THE ESSENTIAL cTBNA BRONCHOSCOPIST©

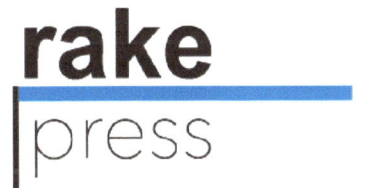

Laguna Beach, CA

The Essential cTBNA Bronchoscopist

Conventional Transbronchial Needle Aspiration

Module 1

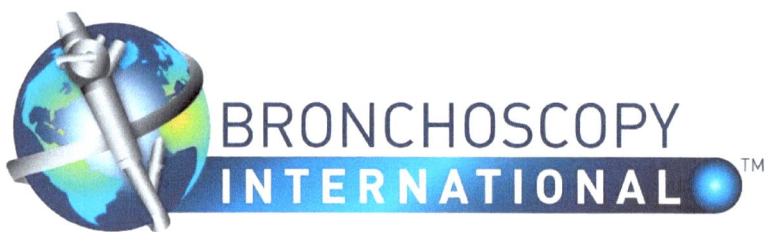

Henri Colt, MD, FCCP, FAWM

With contributions from Drs. Septimiu Murgu, Grigoris Stratakos, Nikos Koufos, Patricia Vujacich and Hernan Iannella

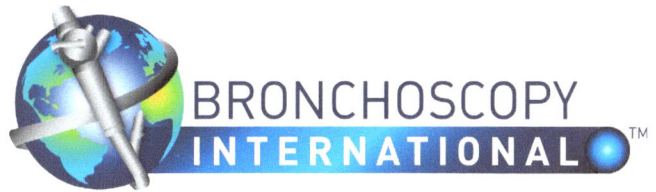

This module was specifically designed for training in conventional transbronchial needle aspiration (cTBNA). The module and its post-test, as well as accompanying interactive Powerpoint© presentations are part of a multidimensional curriculum that includes step-by-step hands-on instruction, simulation, instructional videos, patient-based practical approach exercises, and didactic lectures.

This educational program has been designed in collaboration with the following members of the Bronchoscopy International team:

Dr. Patricia Vujacich (Buenos Aires, Argentina)

Dr. Pedro Garcia Mantilla (Lima, Peru)

Dr. Grigoris Stratakos (Athens, Greece)

Dr. Nikos Koufos (Athens, Greece)

Dr. Hernan Iannella (Buenos Aires, Argentina)

rake
press

Bronchoscopy International, Laguna Beach, CA 92651

Colt Henri G

The Essential cTBNA Bronchoscopist© First Edition, 2015

From, The Essential Bronchoscopist Series™

Title 1: The Essential cTBNA Bronchoscopist; Pulmonary diseases; Thoracic medicine

ISBN-13: 978-1517342692 ISBN-10: 1517342694

1. The Essential Flexible Bronchoscopist©
2. The Essential EBUS Bronchoscopist©
3. The Essential cTBNA Bronchoscopist©
4. The Essential Intensivist Bronchoscopist
5. The Essential Interventional Bronchoscopist
6. The Essential of Bronchoscopy Education©

Manufactured in the United States of America

1 2 3 4 5 6 7 8 9 10

FIRST EDITION

The Essential cTBNA Bronchoscopist

conventional transbronchial needle aspiration

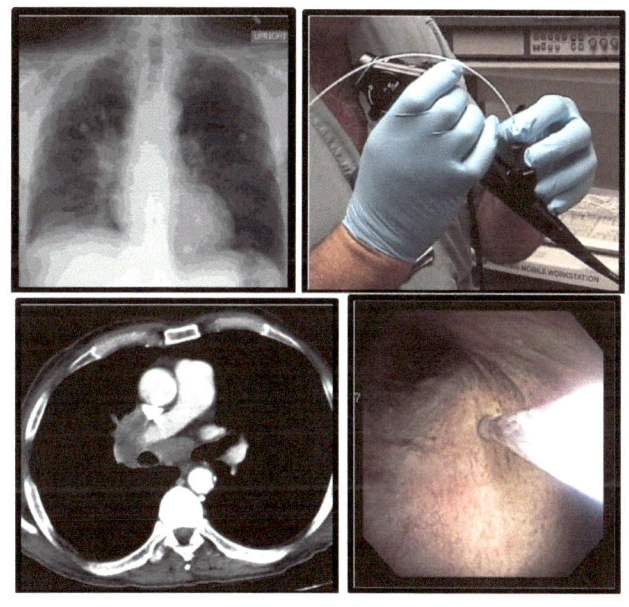

Henri Colt MD

With S. Murgu, G. Stratakos, N. Koufos, P. Vujacich, and H. Iannella

THE ESSENTIAL BRONCHOSCOPIST™ SERIES

Funding statement

Funding for The Essential cTBNA Bronchoscopist© is a result of collaborative work among members of Bronchoscopy International, The Argentine Association for Bronchology, and the bronchoscopy group of the Hellenic Thoracic Society. No corporate support was either solicited or received for this work.

Copyright statement

Essential cTBNA Bronchoscopist© Disclaimer

Acknowledgements

We thank all those who have contributed to the art and science of conventional TBNA and who have helped promote the use of this essential minimally invasive procedure around the world. Particular thanks to Drs. Stefano Gasparini, Hideo Saka, Artemio Garcia, and to the dozens of physicians who espouse Bronchoscopy International's philosophy of an "education without borders."

The Essential Conventional TBNA Bronchoscopist

Conventional transbronchial needle aspiration

TABLE OF CONTENTS

§

MODULE 1

THIRTY MULTIPLE CHOICE QUESTION/ANSWER SETS

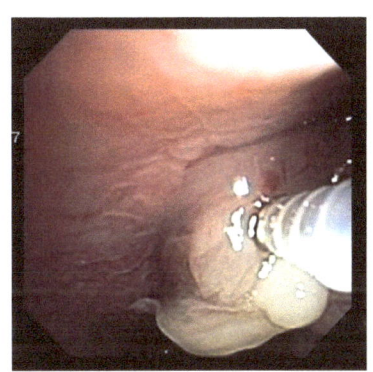

The Essential cTBNA Bronchoscopist MODULE 1

LEARNING OBJECTIVES

After completing this module the reader should be able to:

1. Describe three specific indications for cTBNA in managing patients with lung disorders.
2. Describe the specific locations of lymph node stations 7, 4R and 4L as well as needle insertion sites to sample these lymph node territories.
3. Describe major vascular anatomic structures that are adjacent to lymph node stations 7, 4R and 4L.
4. Describe three different cTBNA techniques (jab, piggyback, and needle to hub).
5. Describe ways to protect the flexible bronchoscope from needle-induced damage.
6. List at least four different complications from cTBNA
7. Specify the role and expected yield of cTBNA among and compared with other diagnostic bronchoscopic procedures.
8. List three major factors that may improve or decrease the quality of cytology smears after cTBNA nodal sampling.

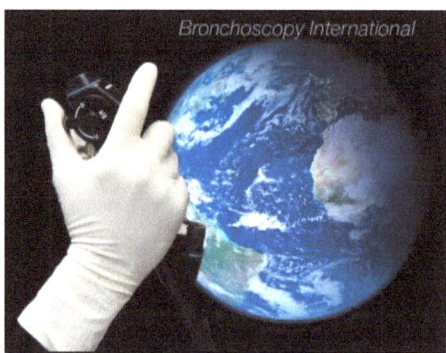

Question I.1 The right pulmonary artery is most adjacent to the anterior wall of the right main bronchus at:

A. The level of the carina near the origin of the right main bronchus.

B. The level of the right upper lobe bronchial orifice and origin of the bronchus intermedius.

C. The origin of the right lower lobe bronchus above the origin of the superior segmental bronchus.

Answer: B

At the level of the orifice of the right upper lobe bronchus, needle insertion through the anterior wall of the right main bronchus risks entering the right pulmonary artery, which lies immediately anterior to the bronchus at this level. Note that the right upper lobe bronchus in this cast is more vertical than usual.

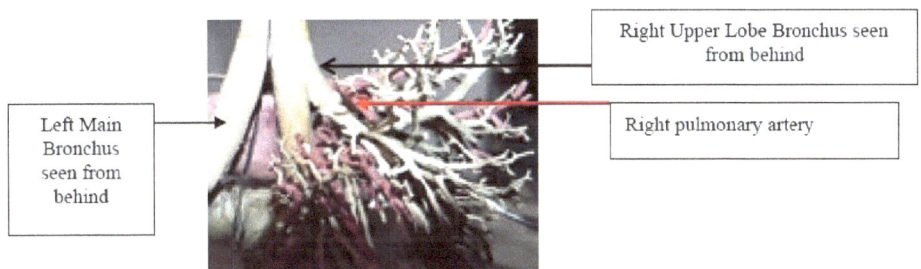

Left Main Bronchus seen from behind

Right Upper Lobe Bronchus seen from behind

Right pulmonary artery

Question I.2 Which of the following statements about the right upper lobe bronchus is correct?

    A. The posterior portion of the right upper lobe bronchus is devoid of any vascular relationships.

    B. The anterior portion of the right upper lobe bronchus is devoid of any vascular relationships.

    C. The pulmonary vein is in direct contact with the right upper lobe bronchus.

Answer: A

No vascular structure is directly adjacent to the posterior aspect of the right upper lobe bronchus. Anterior lies the pulmonary vein, but it is not in direct contact with the bronchus. The right pulmonary artery is adjacent to the anterior wall of the right upper lobe bronchus and origin of the bronchus intermedius. Needle aspiration at this site would be dangerous. Note that the direction of the right upper lobe bronchus in this cast is more vertical than usual.

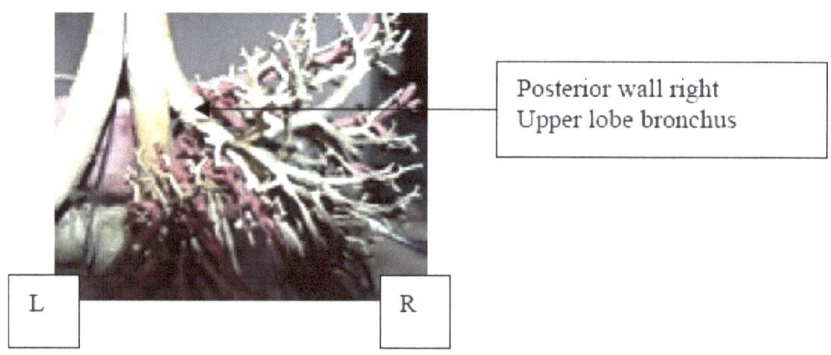

Question I.3 While performing transbronchial needle aspiration of nodal station 4R (right paratracheal), you insert the needle 2 cm above the carina, and laterally at the 3 o'clock position (imagining the interior of the airway as a clock face and using the carina as the central reference point). Which of the following is a major anatomic danger?

A. The aorta

B. The right pulmonary artery

C. The azygos vein

D. The esophagus

Answer: C

Anterior and to the right of the distal third of the trachea lie the superior vena cava and the azygos vein. Needle insertion at this site risks causing pneumothorax or bleeding. The right pulmonary artery is anterior to the right main bronchus and origin from the right upper lobe bronchus. Needle insertion through the anterior wall of the right main bronchus at the level of the origin of the right upper lobe bronchus should be avoided. The esophagus lies closely (within 2-3 mm) behind the posterior wall of the trachea and left main bronchus. The innominate artery and the aortic arch lie directly anterior to the trachea, just above the main carina and coursing slightly to the left of the distal trachea where one can see a slight indent and faint pulsations. Obviously, it would be unwise to insert a needle into this area!

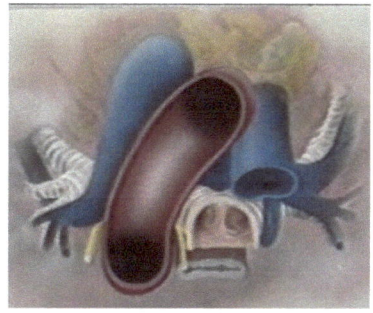

Question I.4 During transbronchial needle aspiration of mediastinal lymphadenopathy, which of the following is most likely to help increase diagnostic yield?

    A. Performing needle aspiration before airway examination or acquisition of other samples.

    B. Maintaining suction during needle withdrawal from the lymph node.

    C. Rinsing the working channel of the bronchoscope before needle insertion.

    D. Asking the cytopathologist to be present to immediately examine the specimens.

Answer: D

Several studies have shown that Rapid OnSite Examination of cTBNA specimens by a trained cytopathologist (ROSE) improves diagnostic yield. In addition, this might allow the bronchoscopist to perform fewer needle passes, and might make additional specimens such as biopsies or brushing less necessary. Most experts recommend rinsing the working channel prior to performing needle aspiration. In addition, in order to avoid false positive results, needle aspiration should be performed prior to airway inspection or biopsies of endobronchial abnormalities. Once the needle (ususally 22G cytology needle) is inserted through the airway wall and into the tumor or lymph node, suction is applied to obtain the sample. Suction should be released prior to removing the needle from the tumor or lymph node in order to avoid avoid contamination from bronchial wall tissue. The bronchoscope should not be connected to wall suction until all needle aspiration samples have been obtained. Using a larger histology needle (19G) might result in greater yield, especially for diagnosis of lymphoma.

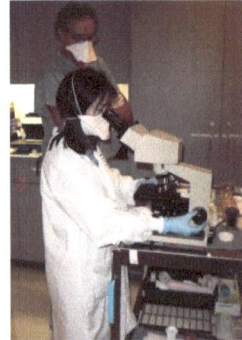

Question I.5 Where are the right paratracheal lymph nodes (IASLC station 4R) in relation to the trachea?

A. Posterior-lateral

B. Anterior-lateral

C. Lateral

D. Posterior

Answer: B

Nodal station 4R is anterolateral to the trachea, and can be accessed by needle aspiration at a site that is two-four intercartilaginous spaces above the carina, aiming the needle anterolaterally towards the 1 or 2 o'clock position (imagining the interior of the airway as a clock face and using the carina as the central reference point). Aiming the needle more laterally risks puncturing the azygos vein. The paratracheal lymph nodes are generally located slightly lateral to the trachea. They are difficult to access because of the very lateral position required of the needle and of the tip of the flexible bronchoscope, especially on the left (station 4L or aortopulmonary window node).

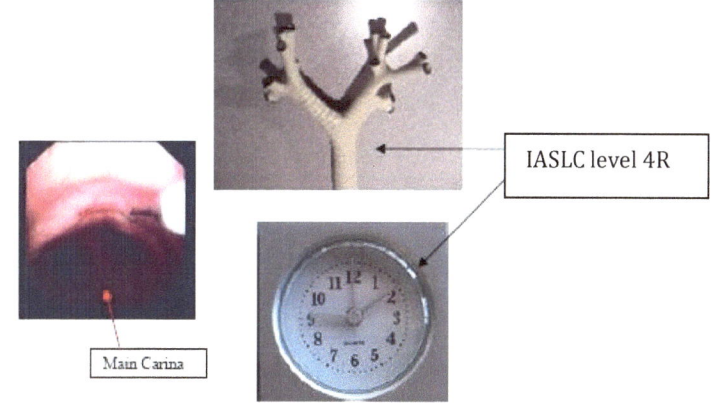

Question I.6 Imagining the interior of the airway as a clock face and using the carina as the central reference point, transbronchial needle aspiration at the 9 o'clock position along the medial wall of the bronchus intermedius at a level just proximal to the right middle lobe bronchial orifice will sample:

    A. The right lower hilar lymph node.

    B. The sub-subcarina lymph node.

    C. The right main bronchus lymph node.

    D. The sub carina lymph node.

Answer: B

The sub-subcarina lymph node is part of an older nomenclature, and is now generally referred to as part of the IASLC level 7 (subcarina) lymph node region. The territory is located between the bronchus intermedius and the left main bronchus, at or near the level of the right middle lobe bronchus. Overall, the level 7 subcarina lymph node region extends caudally to the lower border of the bronchus intermedius on the right, and caudally to the upper border of the left upper lobe bronchus on the left. In order to sample this territory, the needle should be inserted directly through or adjacent to the carina in order to sample nodes directly below the bifurcation, or at the 3 o'clock position along the medial wall of the right main bronchus, just proximal to the level of the right upper lobe bronchial orifice (if the bronchoscopist is standing in front of or to the side of the patient), or at the 9 o' clock position along the medial wall of the right main bronchus (if the operator is standing at the head of the patient).

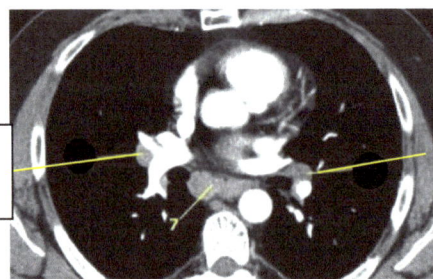

| Interobar nodes | Interlobar nodes |
| IASLC 11R inferior | IASLC 11L |

Aortic arch

Needle through bifurcation

Pulmonary artery

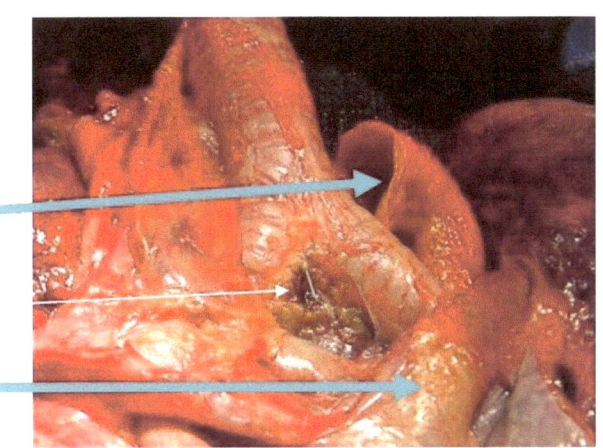

IASLC level 7

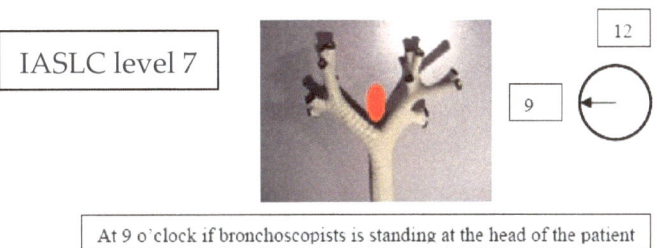

At 9 o'clock if bronchoscopists is standing at the head of the patient

Question I.7 When performing transbronchial or transcarinal needle aspiration, which of the following appears to be most important for increasing diagnostic yield?

A. Performing up to 7 passes with the cytology needle.

B. Performing ROSE (rapid onsite examination) of cTBNA specimens.

C. Using the largest and stiffest needle possible.

D. Obtaining the needle specimen after bronchoalveolar washings or biopsies.

Answer: B

The mean yield of cTBNA is 70-80% in case of lung cancer (sensitivity ranging from 37%-89% with a specificity of 96%), and may be as high as 90% in benign diseases such as sarcoidosis with a recent metanalysis of 21 studies showing a pooled yield of 62%. Yield is increased when cytopathologists can immediately determine whether samples are representative (ROSE). This is standard of practice and should be encouraged in institutions where cTBNA is performed. Needle aspiration should be performed BEFORE other specimens are collected in order to avoid contamination and false positives. While the stiffer, larger-bore, two part histology needle appears helpful for transcarinal sampling, it is more technically challenging to insert through the working channel of the flexible bronchoscope and may be impossible to use in more distal airways. Most investigators find that at least 3-5 needle passes are necessary to make a diagnosis, after which diagnostic yield increases very slightly to 7 passes. Experts agree that cTBNA sensitivity is affected by operator skill and experience, the location and nature of the lesion being sampled (level 4R and 7 provide the greatest yield), the number of aspirates, and the prevalence of malignancy. Yield is also increased when the lesion sampled is larger.

References:

1. Huang JA, Browning R, and Wang KP. Counterpoint: Should endobronchial ultrasound guide veery transbronchial needle aspiration of lymph nodes? No. Chest 2013;144:734-736.
2. Agarwall R et al. efficacy and safety of conventional transbronchial needle aspiration in sarcoidosis. Respir Care 2013;58:683-693.

Question I.8 Which of the following known complications of bronchoscopic needle aspiration can be avoided if proper technique is used?

    A. Hemomediastinum

    B. Pneumothorax

    C. Bronchial hemorrhage

    D. Fracture of needle catheter

    E. Bacterial pericarditis

Answer: D

Proper technique, training, and practice should prevent fracture of the needle catheter by the needle during use. In addition, proper technique will also prevent harming the working channel of the bronchoscope with a protruding needle tip. The needle should never be withdrawn or inserted into the bronchoscope without first ensuring that the needle is well within the catheter. Other complications of needle aspiration such as those listed above occur rarely and are probably unavoidable. Significant bleeding after needle aspiration occurs rarely, even when vascular puncture is confirmed by bloody return in the syringe or catheter during suctioning. Other suggestions to avoid scope damage during cTBNA are (1) to always assure that the beveled edge of the needle is inside the distal metal hub before removing the needle, (2) to avoid mocing the needle proximal to the metal hub so that the needle cannot accidently perforate the plastic catheter, (3) to keep the proximal and distal ends of the flexible bronchoscope scope at the time of needle insertion and removal, (4) to avoid advancing the needle if resistance is encountered, (5) to avoid advancing the needle out of the catheter until the distal end of the cather is outside of the distal end of the flexible bronchoscope. Good communication with the bronchoscopy assistant is essential for a safe and effective procedure.

Question I.9 In regards to transbronchial needle aspiration, which of the following has the greatest risk of damaging the flexible bronchoscope?

   A. Jabbing method for needle penetration.
   B. Piggyback method for needle penetration.
   C. Hub against wall method for needle penetration.
   D. Use of a nonretractable needle.
   E. Cough method for needle penetration.

Answer: D

Using a nonretractable needle or a needle-catheter ensemble that has been damaged such that the needle cannot be retracted into its catheter is most likely to damage the working channel of a flexible bronchoscope. The other methods are each useful for penetrating through the airway wall. While keeping the bronchoscope as straight as possible, and with the bending tip in a neutral position, the retracted needle catheter ensemble is advanced through the working channel of the bronchoscope. The needle is advanced and locked into place after the metal hub is visible beyond the tip of the scope. The catheter is retracted and the scope is advanced to the target area. With the "jabbing method", the needle is thrust through the intercartilaginous space using a quick firm jab to the catheter while the scope is held at the nose or mouth. The "hub method" has the needle in the retracted position so that the distal end (metal hub) of the catheter is placed in direct contact with the airway wall, and held firmly while the needle is pushed out of the catheter and through the airway wall. The "piggyback method" has the catheter fixed against the proximal end of the instrument insertion port (using either an index finger or with the help of an assistant). This is done after the needle has been advanced and locked into position at the target site. The bronchoscope and the needle-catheter ensemble are then advanced together until the entire needle penetrates the airway wall. With the "cough method" the bronchoscopist first employs the piggyback or jabbing technique. The needle is placed directly against the target area and the patient is asked to cough. The cough forces the needle through the airway wall. Once the needle is inside the target, it should be moved forward and backward while suction is maintained in order to shear off cells. Suction is then released, the tip of the bronchoscope is straightened if necessary, the needle is withdrawn from the target, retracted into its catheter and the needle-catheter ensemble is withdrawn from the scope.

Question I.10 After performing transbronchial needle aspiration, the needle cannot be withdrawn into its catheter. You should:

A. Pull the needle completely into the working channel of the scope anyway in order to remove it.

B. Straighten the bronchoscope. Then remove the needle and the flexible bronchoscope simultaneously while keeping it in the middle of the airway but without pulling the needle back into the working channel of the scope.

C. Straighten the bronchoscope. Pull the needle into the working channel so that only the tip of the needle is visible beyond the tip of the scope. Then remove the needle and the flexible bronchoscope simultaneously while keeping it in the middle of the airway.

D. Straighten the bronchoscope. Then pull the needle back into the working channel in order to remove it.

Answer: C

It is safest to straighten the bronchoscope, and while keeping the needle tip in view, to pull the entire ensemble out. By keeping the scope and needle tip in the middle of the airway, there is no risk of injury the airway mucosa. The only danger is to scratch pharyngeal or nasal mucosa. This risk is minimal if the scope is "straight" and without distal flexion or extension, and if only a small portion of the needle tip is visible beyond the distal tip of the bronchoscope.

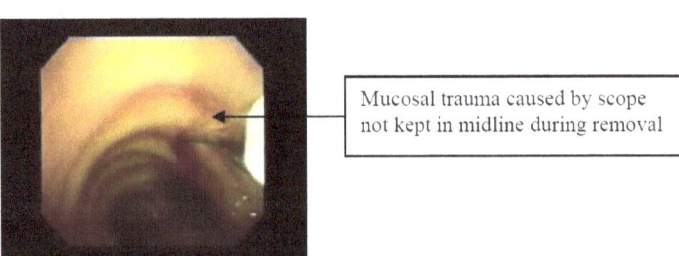

Mucosal trauma caused by scope not kept in midline during removal

Question I.11 A patient with subcarinal adenopathy undergoes flexible bronchoscopy and transcarinal needle aspiration. The cytopathologist is present on site to inform you that the first pass (shown in the Figure below) has no material in it. The second pass could be made:

A. 3-5 mm below on either side of the carina in an infero-medial direction.

B. One intercartilaginous space above and directed more anterior.

C. Two intercartilaginous spaces above and in an anterolateral direction.

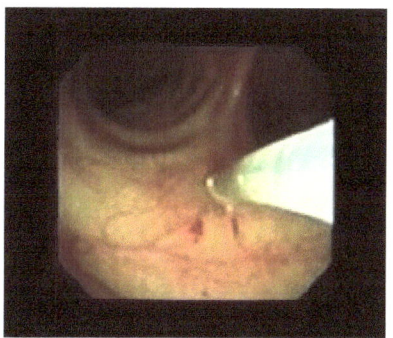

Answer: A

Subcarinal lymph nodes (station 7) can be sampled by inserting the needle directly through the main carina in an inferior direction, or by inserting the needle 3-4 mm below on either side of the carina, directing the needle inferiorly and medially. If the needle were directed more superiorly, anteriorly and laterally (answer c) the 4R region would be sampled. If the needle were directed more superiorly and anteriorly (answer b) the anterior portion of station 7 would be sampled. If the needle were directed posterior, the posterior portion of station 7 could be sampled (but this also risks causing pneumothorax because of proximity of the azygoesophageal recess). While any tumors may eventually involve subcarina lymph nodes, this region is the primary drainage area for primary lung cancers originating in the right middle lobe, right lower lobe, left lower lobe, and left upper lobe lingular segment. Right upper lobe tumors drain primarily to the right paratracheal (4R) region. Left upper division tumors drain primarily to the left subaortic, hilar and intrapulmonary nodes.

IASLC station 7

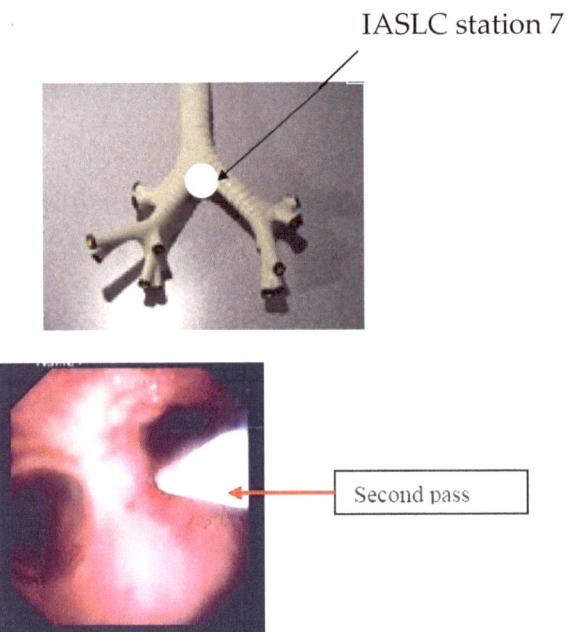

Second pass

Question I.12 Flexible bronchoscopy with transbronchial needle aspiration of a left upper lobe abnormality is performed in a 33-year-old patient with Acquired Immune Deficiency Syndrome (AIDS). After the procedure, the technician notices that the leak test is positive. An air leak is detected from the surface of the flexible bronchoscope. He asks you for instructions. You should tell him to:

A. Disinfect the scope in a Glutaraldehyde bath before packing it and sending it to the manufacturer for repair.

B. Clean only the working channel with warm water and detergent, then pack the scope and send it to the manufacturer for repair.

C. To not clean the bronchoscope at all. Place the bronchoscope in a biohazard bag.

D. Pack the scope and send it to the manufacturer with a note explaining the circumstances of scope damage.

E. Continue with manual cleaning of the bronchoscope and all internal channels using only warm water and detergent, then pack it in a biohazard bag and send it to the manufacturer for repair.

Answer: C

A leak test should be routinely performed after cTBNA to assure that the bronchoscope has not been damaged during the procedure. Bronchoscopes should not be submerged in fluid until a leak test has been performed. If the leak test is positive, water or fluid immersion risks serious and costly damage to the bronchoscope. The bronchoscope will need to be sent out for repair. Universal precautions should be routinely followed in order to prevent the transmission of infection. The patient's known AIDS infection is therefore irrelevant.

Question I.13 A 71 year old Chinese woman presented to the outpatient clinic with weight loss and a chronic cough of 3 months' duration. Her medical history included hypertension and hemithyroidectomy 20 years ago for Graves' disease. Chest radiograph revealed a left paratracheal mass with contralateral tracheal deviation. A chest computed tomography scan revealed retrosternal goiter with an enlarged left lower paratracheal lymph node. A possible next step is to:

A. Perform thyroid function tests for this likely benign disorder

B. Proceed with open mediastinal exploration.

C. Proceed with cTBNA of the left lower paratracheal lymph node.

D. Proceed with CT guided transthoracic needle aspiration of the thyroid mass.

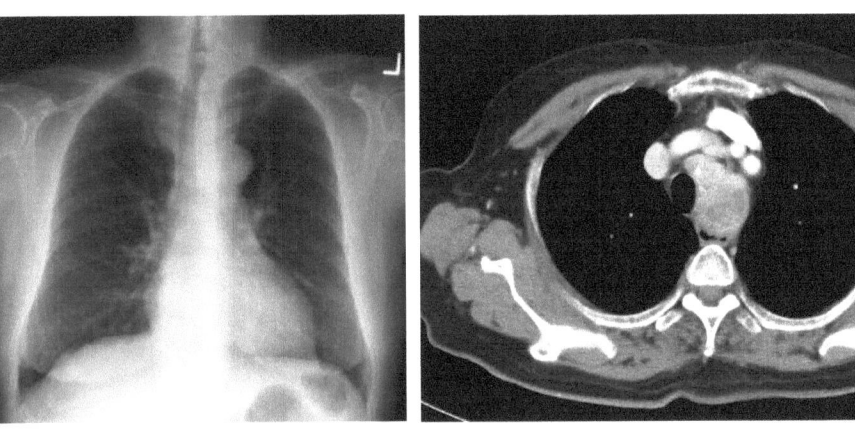

Answer: C

Mediastinal goitres represent about 10% of mediastinal masses. Computed tomography findings include encapsulation, lobulation, heterogeneity, and continuity between cervical and mediastinal components. While thyroid function tests should be performed, histologic diagnosis is warranted because malignancy develops in a number of mediastinal goiters. cTBNA represents an alternative to percutaneous needle aspiration or open surgical exploration.

Proposed indications include staging the radiologically normal mediastinum in suspected or confirmed lung cancer, mediastinal restaging after induction chemotherapy, and diagnosis of mediastinal, hilar, peribronchial, paratracheal, or intrapulmonary masses. In this case, needle aspiration of the lymph node as well as of the retrosternal goiter revealed clusters of follicular cells consistent with benign thyroid tissue. It is noteworthy that cTBNA of high paratracheal lymph nodes and paratracheal lesions can be difficult. In most cases today, operators prefer using EBUS-guided TBNA if available in such instances. Furthermore, because cTBNA is essentially a "blind" technique, there is no way to determine whether samples are coming from necrotic or non-necrotic target areas, which might affect diagnostic yield and diminish (in case only areas of necrosis are sampled) overall sensitivity of the procedure. Larger 19G histology needles have been shown to increase diagnostic yield as compared to smaller 22 G cytology needles in several studies (sometimes by up to 35%), but it can be more difficult to pass the histology needle through the working channel of the flexible bronchoscope, and its use may not be possible in every patient. When used, the histology needle allows retrieval of core specimens, which may be particularly important to increase yield in patients with benign diseases such as tuberculosis or histoplasmosis, sarcoidosis, or in patients with suspected or known lymphoma, lung cancer, or metastatic cancers involving mediastinal lymph nodes.

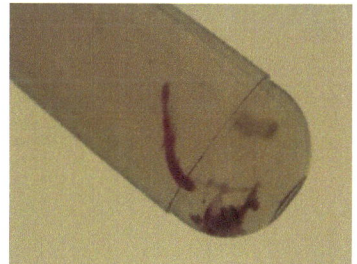

Question I.14 A patient with a right upper lobe mass underwent an integrated PET-CT (see Image) which showed a PET positive level 11R and PET negative level 7 and level 4L (not shown) lymph nodes. After white light bronchoscopy revealed no endobronchial abnormalities, you proceed with cTBNA for diagnosis and staging. The first thing you should do is:

    A. Sample station 7 because the diagnostic yield is higher than from station 10R.

    B. Sample station 11R because it is PET positive.

    C. Evaluate and sample left sided mediastinal lymph nodes, if present.

    D. Evaluate and sample any pre-carinal lymph nodes, if present.

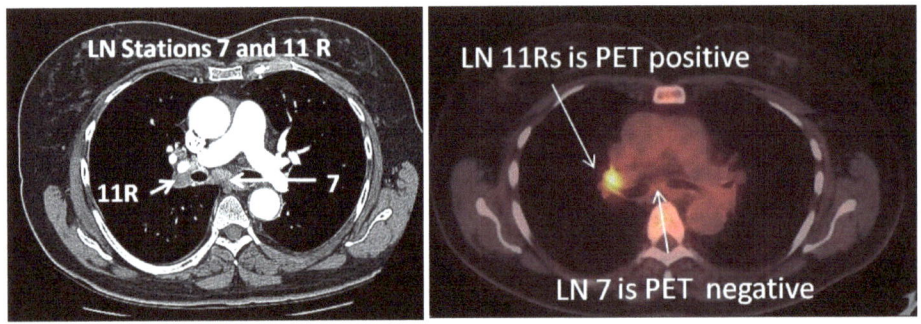

Answer: C

Overall, the cTBNA diagnostic yield is higher from subcarinal nodes than from other stations. This would argue for initially sampling the subcarinal node. However, selecting the PET positive node for cTBNA could increase the sensitivity of the procedure. When performed for diagnosis and staging purposes, however, cTBNA should be performed first from N3 nodes, followed by N2 nodes and for diagnosis, when necessary, N1 nodes. If N3 nodes were found to be positive for malignancy on rapid on-site cytological evaluation, the procedure could be terminated. In this case N3 nodes are the contralateral (left) sided mediastinal nodes. The pre-carinal nodes are part of station 4R, thus in this case, are still N2 nodes.

Question I.15 Which of the following statements about cTBNA smears is FALSE?

A. A delay in processing a cTBNA sample may hinder the process of smearing.

B. Air drying artifacts and bubbles on the slide can cause uneven distiribution of the material being smeared.

C. After placing the specimen on the slide, smear it to produce a thin layer that uniformly distributes the specimen on the slide.

D. A thick smear may cause stucked and overlapping cells.

E. While performing the smear, applying excessive force between two slides provides a better distribution of the material on the slides.

Answer: E

Applying excessive force between two slides does not necesseraly distribute better the material on the slide. On the contrary, diagnostic material can be completely destroyed when this technique is applied. The distribution of the material should be done smoothly so that it can be done equally on the slide and at the same time cellular components remain intact. Any delay in processing the sample may result in coagulation inside the needle lumen or on the slide surface and hinder the process of smearing. Particularly when Diff-Quick stain is used the quantity of sample fluid must be just enough to smear, enabling it to dry as soon as possible. Presence of bubbles on the slide can cause uneven distribution of the material. In terms of quantity, only a small drop of sample should be adequate and can help to avoid overlapping cells.

References

1. H. Colt, S. Murgu, Bronchoscopy and Central Airway Disorders, A patient-centered approach. Elsevier-Saunders, 2012.

2. Centikaya et al. Diagnostic value of transbronchial needle aspiration by Wang 22-gauge cytology needle in intrathoracic lymphadenopathy. Chest. 2004;125:527-531.

Question I.16 While performing cTBNA from a subcarinal lymph node (level 7), you obtain a bloody sample. This could be caused by which of the the following?

    A. The left atrium has been pentrated.

    B. The right pulmonary artery has been penetrated.

    C. The inferior pulmonary vein has been penetrated.

    D. A blood vessel within the lymph node itself has been penetrated.

    E. All of the above.

Answer: E

Each of the anatomic structures listed: left atrium, right pulmonary artery and inferior pulmonary vein could be inadevertently penetrated during cTBNA of a level 7 node. Keep in mind that blood vessels inside a lymph node are not uncommon. The use of EBUS-TBNA alows direct visualization of the node during needle insertion, as well as identification of blood vessels as hypoechoic structures that are Doppler positive (see Image).

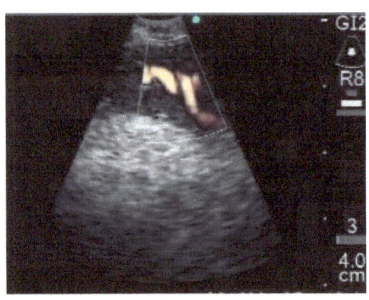

Question I.17 After two aspirates from the subcarinal lymph node in a patient with suspected lung cancer, the cytologist tells you that the Diff-Quick stain shows scant lymphocytes and benign bronchial cells. You should:

A. Continue the procedure and perform another one or two aspirates.

B. Abort the procedure and wait for the final results.

C. Abort the procedure since the specimen shows lymphocytes.

D. Continue the procedure until a diagnosis is obtained.

Answer: A

A cytology specimen is considered adequate or representative if there is presence of frankly malignant cell, granulomas or lymphocytes, lymphoid tissue, or clusters of anthracotic pigment-laden macrophages. Higher yields may be obtained by obtaining aspirates from the periphery of the node. Therefore, the procedure should be continued and another one or two aspirates should be performed with the intent to sample other regions of the lymph node. Aborting the procedure because lymphocytes are seen and assuming the specimen is representative is premature. The specimen is considered inadequate or non-representative if there are no cellular components, scant lymphocytes (defined as <40 per HPF), blood only, cartilage or bronchial epithelial cells only. A quantitative cut-off value of at least 30% cellularity composed of lymphocytes has been arbitrarily proposed by some experts. There is a good correlation between rapid on-site evaluation and the final cytologic diagnosis, so aborting the procedure hoping that the final results will be diagnostic is not an appropriate next step. However, during cTBNA the diagnostic yield plateaus after 3 to 5 passes. Therefore continuing the procedure "indefinitely" thinking that eventually a diagnosis will be made is also not warranted and may increase the risk for complications from prolonged sedation, anesthesia, or procedure related complications such as pneumothorax, bleeding, bacteremia, pericarditis, mediastinitis, or scope breakage.

References

1. Alsharif M, Andrade RS, Groth SS et al. Endobronchial ultrasound-guided transbronchial fine needle aspiration: the University of Minnesota experience, with emphasis on usefulness, adequacy assessment, and diagnostic difficulties. Am J Clin Pathol 2008;130: 434-443.

2. Lee HS, Lee GK, Lee HS et al. Real-time endobronchial ultrasound guided transbronchial needle aspiration in mediastinal staging of nonsmall cell lung cancer: how many aspirations per target lymph node station. Chest 2008;134:368-374.

3. Trisolini R, Lazzari A, Patelli. Conventional vs endobronchial ultrasound-guided transbronchial needle aspiration of the mediastinum. Chest 2004;126:1005-1006.

4. Diacon AH, Schuurmans J, Theron K et al. Transbronchial needle aspirations: how many passes per target site? Eur Respir J 2007;29:357-362.

Question I.18 While performing cTBNA from a large right lower pretracheal node in an asymptomatic 30 year old non-smoking African American woman, the cytologist tells you that there is «non-caseating granulomatous inflammation». Based on this information, which of the following is the most likely diagnosis?

  A. Primary lung carcinoma

  B. Sarcoidosis

  C. Tuberculosis

  D. Lymphoma

Answer: B

This patient has a high pre-test probability for sarcoidosis (non-smoking African American female under 50 years). In sarcoidosis, lymph node enlargement is usually seen in the right paratracheal, aorto-pulmonary window and hilar regions. The cytology specimens when used in conjuction with clinical findings, radiological and laboratory investigations, is a useful tool in the diagnosis of sarcoidosis. In patients with granulomatous disease, cTBNA and endobronchial ultrasound guided (EBUS-TBNA) are of great value. In a randomized study with Sarcoidosis patients, EBUS-TBNA was found to have the highest diagnostic yield when combined with transbronchial lung biopsy, but on the other hand the diagnostic yield of cTBNA plus endobronchial biopsy (EBB) and TBLB was found similar. Demonstration of granulomas remains an essential criterion, but as granulomatous inflammation can be seen in host of conditions, it is necessary to exclude all possible cause, as well as to correlate with other findings, before arriving at the diagnosis of sarcoidosis. One should keep in mind that lymph nodes harboring both necrotizing and non-necrotizing granulomas and malignancy have been described[2,3]. In general, to establish a diagnosis of sarcoidosis it is necessary that granulomata must be present in two or more organs, with no agent known to cause a granulomatous response being identified. A search should be made for other causes of granulomatous inflammation, including mycobacteria, fungi, parasites, and foreign bodies. Tuberculosis may also present as non-caseating granulomas and, if suspected, the specimen should be also sent for culture. One major pitfall may be finding non-caseating granulomas in sarcoid reaction. These are morphologically identical to the granulomas of sarcoidosis. Sarcoid reactions have been reported in patients with various lymphomas, non-small cell carcinoma of the lung, and germ cell carcinoma, either in lymph nodes draining the malignancy or in remote lymph node stations[4]. These sarcoid-like granulomas appear to represent a local T cell-mediated immune reaction. The diagnosis of lymphoma may be controversial, although the use of flow cytometry, molecular biology techniques and immunocytochemistry on cell block preps may provide enough information for a definitive diagnosis or robust data for a diagnosis of lymphoma without any further specification.

References

1. Gupta D, Dadhwal D, Agarwal R, et al. Endobronchial ultrasound-guided transbronchial needle aspiration vs conventional transbronchial needle aspiration in the diagnosis of sarcoidosis. Chest 2014;146:547-556.

2. Pandey M, Abraham EK, Chandramohan K, et al. Tuberculosis and metastatic carcinoma coexistence in axillary lymph node: a case report. World J Surg Oncol 2003;1:3.

3. Laurberg P. Sarcoid reactions in pulmonary neoplasms. Scand J Respir Dis 1975;56:20-27.

4. Steinfort DP, Irving LB. Sarcoid reactions in regional lymph nodes of patients with non-small cell lung cancer: Incidence and implications for minimally invasive staging with endobronchial ultrasound. Lung Cancer 2009;66:305-308.

Question I.19 A patient is referred for EBUS-TBNA from the subcarinal lymph node. The CT scan is shown below. Your EBUS scope is out for repair and expected to be returned in several days. The patient and his referring doctor would like to proceed with a diagnostic intervention as soon as possible. What is the most appropriate next step?

- A. Wait until the EBUS scope is available and then proceed with EBUS-TBNA.
- B. Refer the patient to your gastroenterologist colleague for EUS-FNA.
- C. Refer the patient to your thoracic surgery colleague for mediastinoscopy.
- D. Proceed with cTBNA with rapid on-site examination.

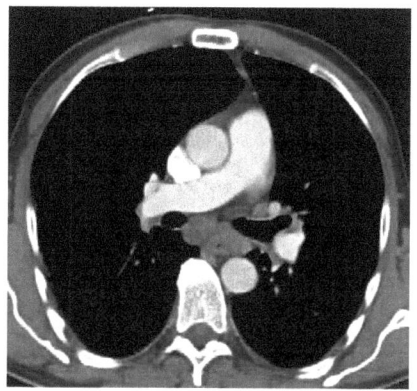

Answer: D

One could argue that waiting for the EBUS scope is appropriate. If diagnosed with lung cancer, this would be a stage IIIA (with bulky lymphadenopathy) and the patient will likely initiate multimodality treatment rather than undergo primary surgical resection. Delaying diagnosis for several days will not impact management. Both the patient and the referring physician, however, wish to obtain a diagnosis as soon as possible. EUS-FNA and mediastinoscopy have a high diagnostic yield for subcarinal lymph nodes, but might delay the diagnosis because necessary specialist consultations may not always be readily available; furthermore, mediastinoscopy is more invasive and with higher complication rates than needle aspiration techniques (if one excludes possible false-negative EBUS-TBNA as a complication). cTBNA with rapid on site examination is an appropriate next step in this patient if diagnosis is rapidly desired. This patient has no other lymph nodes visible on computed tomography. The yield of cTBNA for large subcarinal lymph nodes is similar to that of EBUS-TBNA. In all other cases (except 4R in some studies), EBUS guidance significantly increases the yield compared with cTBNA.

References

1. Herth F, Becker H, and Ernst A. Conventional versus ultrasound-guided transbronchial needle aspiration: a randomized trial. Chest 2004;125:322–325.

Question I.20 While performing cTBNA, which of the following can damage the bronchoscope?

A. Improper handling of a transbronchial needle.

B. Attempting to pass an instrument through a fully flexed distal extremity of the bronchoscope

C. Advancing the bronchoscope by pushing down from the handle.

D. Bronchoscopy through an endotracheal tube in a mechanically ventilated patient.

E. All of the above.

Answer: E

In order to avoid damage to the working channel of a bronchoscope, all transbronchial needles should be handled properly. No needle should be inserted or withdrawn if its sharp tip is visible and protruding beyond the protective sheath. Needles should not be inserted forcefully through a flexed bronchoscope when the distal tip is bent at an acute angle because the needle may become caught inside the working channel or perforate the bronchoscope. Advancing the bronchoscope by pushing down on the universal handle (control section) can bend the instrument proximally, making it more difficult to insert instruments through the working channel. Any resistance that is felt as an instrument is passes through the working channel can be a sign that the instrument is scratching, and possibly damaging the inside of the working channel. This is especially the case for transbronchial needles! The bronchoscope should be advanced by moving the entire ensemble (insertion cord and control section) together. Sometimes this can be done by simply leaning forward. It is noteworthy that a flexible bronchoscope can be damaged whenever it is inserted through an endotracheal tube, and that patient can bite down on an endotracheal tube even when the operator things the patient is paralyzed. Paralysis may be incomplete. Other times, bite blockers slip and the endotracheal tube becomes wedged between the teeth. Lubrication with silicone, xylocaine gel, or normal saline solution should be routine before inserting the bronchoscope into the endotracheal tube.

Question I.21 In which of the following conditions cTBNA of an accessible adenopathy is most useful to improve diagnostic yield?

- A. Histoplasma capsulatum infection.
- B. Mycobacterium tuberculosis infection.
- C. Sarcoidosis.
- D. Cryptogenic organizing pneumonia.
- E. Wegener's granulomatosis.

Answer: C

Sarcoidosis remains a diagnosis of exclusion. Sarcoidosis may have several endobronchial appearances, none of which are specific: mucosal nodularity, hypertrophy hyperemia, edema, and bronchial stricture). Small raised whitish lesions can be seen, or mucosa may be granular, firm, erythematous or thickened. Other granulomatous diseases may also have these appearances. Greatest yield for diagnosis is from combined bronchoscopic and endobronchial biopsies. Endobronchial biopsies may contain disease even when the mucosa appears normal bronchoscopically. Transcarinal needle aspiration can also be helpful in patients with mediastinal adenopathy. Since non-caseating granulomas may be found in endobronchial biopsies, transcarinal needle aspiration specimens, and bronchoscopic lung biopsy samples, it appears reasonable to obtain tissue using all methods in an attempt to increase diagnostic yield for this disease. The yield for infectious lung disease using bronchoalveolar lavage alone is excellent, and little is gained by obtaining tissue specimens. In patients with idiopathic interstitial lung diseases or pulmonary vasculitis, endobronchial biopsies or cTBNA findings are too often nonspecific and thoracoscopic lung biopsy may be required in certain cases for satisfactory and definitive tissue diagnosis.

Question I.22 A 39-year-old man with a history of testicular cancer three years ago is now found to have a 4 cm right lower lobe opacity on chest radiograph. Computed tomography scan (see image) reveals that the mass contains calcifications (arrows). The mass is located in the right lower lobe, and is relatively central. Radiographically, there is no endobronchial disease or associated lymphadenopathy. The patient has no symptoms. The case is presented at a weekly chest conference. The medical oncologist fears that the mass is a metastasis. The radiologist is not as certain, but states that the lesion should be accessible by bronchoscopy. The interventional radiologist states the patient has a 30 percent chance for pneumothorax if the lesion is sampled percutaneously using fluoroscopic or computed-tomographic guidance. A thoracic surgeon recommends immediate thoracotomy and lung resection if frozen sections during thoracotomy are positive for malignancy. An inspection flexible bronchoscopy had been performed before the chest conference. No airway abnormalities were seen and only non-diagnostic bronchial washings had been obtained. You would now propose which of the following?

A. Thoracotomy with lower lobectomy.

B. Video-assisted thoracoscopy with needle aspiration under thoracoscopic guidance.

C. Flexible bronchoscopy with fluoroscopic guidance for biopsy or needle sampling of the abnormality and on-site cytopathology.

D. Flexible bronchoscopy with blind transbronchial needle aspiration.

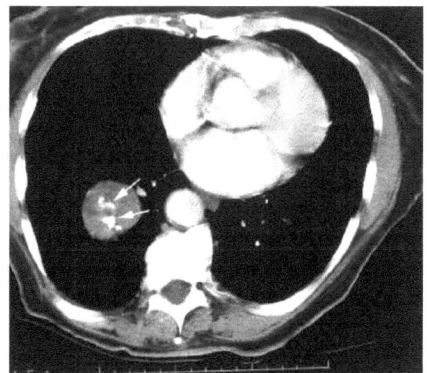

Answer: C

This patient should probably NOT have undergone the "exploratory" flexible bronchoscopy that provided no diagnostic material or useful information for subsequent decision-making, and did cause increased health care expenditures and patient discomfort. It would be unclear why bronchoscopic lung biopsy or needle aspiration would not have been attempted using fluoroscopic guidance. Possible non-bronchoscopic options are to proceed with thoracoscopically guided needle aspiration, percutaneous CT-guided needle aspiration, or percutaneous ultrasound-guided needle aspiration, recognizing there is a risk for pneumothorax because of the location of the abnormality. Other bronchoscopic procedures that could be considered include needle aspiration or biopsy using electronavigation, and needle aspiration or biopsy using small caliber flexible bronchoscopy or guide-sheath. An open thoracotomy can probably be avoided.

Question I.23 During a cTBNA staging procedure in a patient with a left upper lobe mass and lymphadenopathy at level 10L, 7, 4L and 4R, you initially start by sampling which of the following nodes?

A. Station 10L

B. Station 7

C. Station 4L

D. Station 4R

Answer: D

For this patient with a left upper lobe mass, station 10L is an ipsilateral N1 node, and stations 7 and 4L are N2, while station 4R is a contra lateral mediastinal node (N3). cTBNA is performed first from N3 nodes, followed by N2 nodes, and if needed for diagnostic purposes N1 nodes. If N3 nodes were found to be positive for malignancy on rapid on-site cytological evaluation, the procedure could be terminated. At this time, from a staging perspective, determining N1 positivity does not alter therapeutic strategies. No benefit has been shown for providing neoadjuvant chemotherapy to patients with known N1 disease, and patients with N1 lymph node involvement are not denied resection if they have an acceptable risk profile for surgery[1].

References

1. Shrager JB. Mediastinoscopy: Still the Gold Standard. Ann Thorac Surg 2010;89:S2084 –9.

Question I.24 A 72 year-old man was admitted with low-grade fever, cough and dyspnea. His chest CT scan showed diffuse alveolar infiltrates in the right lung and enlarged subcarinal and pretracheal nodes of 2.5 cm and 2.0 cm in diameter respectively. The patient gradually developed severe respiratory insufficiency requiring intubation and mechanical ventilation. In the ICU, a diagnostic bronchoscopy was scheduled in order to perform a bronchoalveolar lavage and cTBNA lymph node sampling. Which of the following statements is TRUE?

A. cTBNA should not be performed in this patient because of the high risk of pneumomediastinum.

B. The bronchoscope/endotracheal tube size ratio is not an important consideration.

C. Frequent suctioning during bronchoscopy is recommended.

D. 100% fraction of inspired O_2 and increased positive-end expiratory pressure (PEEP) are recommended.

E. 100% fraction of inspired O_2 and decreased positive-end expiratory pressure (PEEP) are recommended.

Answer: E

In critically ill patients in the ICU setting, flexible bronchoscopy is often employed to inspect the airways, remove secretions or blood clots, and collect samples for culture. Invasive procedures that can be performed are limited due to increased risk of barotrauma, pneumothorax, hemodynamic instability and coagulopathies. When performing a bronchoscopy, the endotracheal tube/bronchoscope size ratio is important. If the endotracheal tube is smaller than 7.5 mm, the bronchoscope can be difficult to insert. It can be damaged or even lodged within the tube. In an 8.0 mm tube, the bronchoscope can occupy more than half of the effective diameter of the tube, which can lead to increased airway pressure, increased auto-PEEP, reduced tidal volumes, hypoxia and hypercarbia. Prior to and during bronchoscopy, 100% inspired oxygen fraction should be administered and PEEP should be decreased in order to avoid increasing intrinsic PEEP (auto-PEEP). In addition, extremely low tidal volume and significant auto-PEEP may develop unless flow, respiratory rate, mode, and ETT size are carefully selected. Pressure-controlled ventilation mode was found to deliver more volume than volume-controlled mechanical ventilation mode. Excessive suctioning during bronchoscopy in patients under mechanical ventilation can remove as much as 200-300 cc of tidal volume, resulting in subsequent drop in PaO_2 and rise in $PaCO_2$. It is recommended to use short intermittent bursts of suctioning < 3 sec each. Going in and out frequently, giving breaks, and allowing the patient time to enhance ventilate and oxygenate better are also options. Overall, cTBNA has been proven to be a safe and useful minimally invasive technique in the ICU in selected patients receiving mechanical ventilation. It has high sensitivity, specificity, and positive predictive values.

References

1. Farrow S, Farrow C, Soni N, et al. Size matters: choosing the right tracheal tube. Anaesthesia. 2012;67:815-819.

2. Lawson RW, Peters JI, Shelledy DC et al. Effects of fiberoptic bronchoscopy during mechanical ventilation in a lung model. Chest 2000;118:824-831.

3. Snow N, Lucas AE. Bronchoscopy in the critically ill surgical patient. Am Surg 1984;50:441-445.

4. Ghamande S, Rafanan A, Dweik R, et al. Role of transbronchial needle aspiration in patients receiving mechanical ventilation. Chest. 2002;122:985-989.

Question I.25 A 38 year old female patient presents with persistent non-productive cough for the last 3 weeks. On chest CT scan a large (>3 cm in diameter), homogenous non-enhancing lesion in the subcarinal area is noted. A bronchoscopy is scheduled and cTBNA is performed. Serous fluid is aspirated from the nodal area and an acellular smear is prepared. All cultures and cytological exams are negative. The most likely diagnosis is:

A. Non-Hodgkin lymphoma.

B. Tuberculosis infection.

C. Bronchogenic cyst.

D. Mediastinal abscess.

E. Small cell lung cancer.

Answer: C

Bronchogenic cysts are usually thin-walled, single or multiple, and lined with columnar ciliated epithelium of congenital origin derived from the primitive foregut. They are most commonly located in the mediastinum, and 15-20% occur in the lung, located primarily on the right side. They may contain clear or hemorrhagic fluid, proteinaceous mucus, calcium or air. Some bronchogenic cysts are asymptomatic and are incidental findings upon radiography, but most patients present with respiratory distress followed by recurring episodes of cough, stridor, and wheezing. On CT scan bronchogenic cysts usually present as a round, well-circumscribed, usually unilocular mass with smooth outlines. About half of the cysts are homogeneous with a near-water density (usually <20 Hounsfield units [HU] on CT). However, infected cysts that contain proteinaceous material and hemorrhagic cysts can have a more solid appearance (up to 80-90 HU), thereby increasing diagnostic uncertainty. Traditional management of cystic lesions involving the mediastinum or lung parenchyma consists of surgical resection. Endobronchial ultrasound-guided transbronchial needle aspiration (EBUS-TBNA) has been used to successfully treat some bronchogenic cysts. Surgical resection may be required for multiloculated intraparenchymal cysts that cannot be aspirated completely. EBUS guidance helps identify multiloculation and completeness of the aspiration.

References

1. Hong G, Song J, Lee KJ, et al. Bronchogenic cyst rupture and pneumonia after endobronchial ultrasound-guided transbronchial needle aspiration: a case report. Tuberc Respir Dis (Seoul) 2013;74:177–180.

2. Takeda S, Miyoshi S, Minami M, et al. Clinical spectrum of mediastinal cysts. Chest 2003;124:125–132.

3. McAdams HP, Kirejczyk WM, Rosado-de-Christenson ML, et al. Bronchogenic cyst: imaging features with clinical and histopathologic correlation. Radiology 2000;217:441–446.

Question I.26 When would you prefer transbronchial needle aspiration over a biopsy forceps for the diagnosis of an endobronchial lesion?

    A. Presence of fleshy vascular endobronchial growth with high risk of bleeding.

    B. Inadequate tissue sampling due to the presence of excessive necrosis.

    C. Presence of a blood clot over the lesion.

    D. Formation of crush artifacts by flexible bronchoscopy.

    E. All of the above.

Answer: E

cTBNA has an established use and value in the diagnosis of mediastinal and hilar adenopathy. Additionally, it is a useful and safe bronchoscopic technique in the diagnosis of bronchogenic carcinoma. When diagnosing endobronchial lesions, cTBNA can be preferred over forceps biopsy in order to decrease the risk of complications such as bleeding, as well as to increase diagnostic yield. Usually, the needle is inserted into a visible exophytic intrabronchial abnormality, or into a submucosal infiltrating lesion. In these cases, the procedure is often referred to as Endobronchial Needle Aspiration (EBNA). This procedure may be preferred instead of endobronchial forceps biopsy or brushing in several instances. For example, the presence of a fleshy vascular endobronchial growth increases the risk of bleeding when forceps biopsy is used instead of a cTBNA/EBNA. Excessive presence of necrosis or blood clot over the lesion may also make EBNA preferable over forceps biopsy. Furthermore, EBNA obtains specimens without forceps biopsy-related crush artifacts that makes slide interpretation difficult. Several studies show an added benefit of performing endobronchial EBNA instead of or in addition to biopsy and brushing. The goal is to obtain a good cytology or core sample. It may be best, therefore, to enter exophytic intrabronchial tumors as perpendicularly (at 90 degrees) as possible, and to approach submucosal tumors from a 30-45 degree angle, in order to get as deep into the lesions as possible. Diagnostic yield of EBNA in both submucosal and exophytic tumors is often greater than 90%.

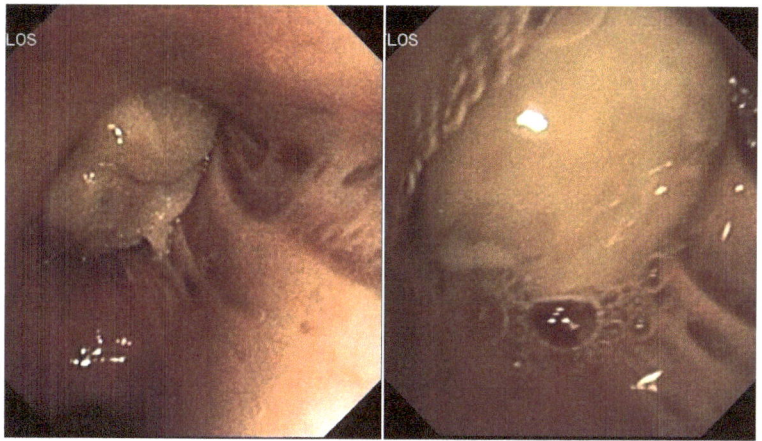

Example of an endobronchial lesion with excessive necrosis present where cTBNA (also called EBNA) should be preferred over biopsy forceps for diagnosis.

References

1. Shital P, Rujuta A, Sanjay M. Transbronchial needle aspiration cytology (TBNA) in endobronchial lesions: a valuable technique during bronchoscopy in diagnosing lung cancer and it will decrease repeat bronchoscopy. J Cancer Res Clin Oncol 2014;140:809-815.

Question I.27 A 42 year old female patient is diagnosed with a solitary pulmonary nodule of 2.8 cm in diameter. The lesion is PET positive, located on the right upper lobe, with bronchus sign on thin-section computed tomography. No lymphadenopathy or distant metastases are noted. A flexible bronchoscopy with endobronchial ultrasonography and fluoroscopy is scheduled. Which of the following statements is TRUE?

A. A bronchial washing is usually adequate for diagnosis.

B. A combined use of transbronchial needle aspiration and transbronchial biopsy can improve the diagnostic yield.

C. The use of transbronchial needle aspiration through the guide sheath should be avoided due to increased risk of complications.

D. Surgery is the only option for diagnosis.

Answer: B

Endobronchial ultrasonography with a guide sheath has improved the diagnostic yield of small-sized peripheral lung lesions. The use of fluoroscopy also helps increase the diagnostic yield and safety of the procedure. The CT bronchus sign is a significant predictive factor for successful bronchoscopic diagnosis. The use of a biopsy forceps for transbronchial biopsies (TBBx) and conventional transbronchial needle aspiration (cTBNA) through the guide sheath are effective and safe procedures for diagnosing peripheral pulmonary lesions. Additionally, cTBNA is more helpful than TBBx when the guide sheath is located outside the lesion. TBBx, cTBNA and transbronchial catheter aspiration are complementary techniques. Combining these three techniques allows specimen collection from small lesions <3 cm in diameter during conventional bronchoscopy.

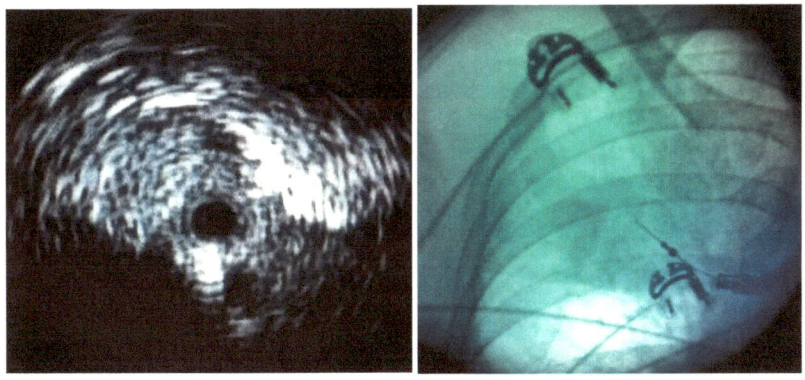

Example of transbronchial needle aspiration through the guiding sheath under endobronchial sonography.

References

1. Franke KJ, Hein M, Domanski U, et al. Transbronchial Catheter Aspiration and Transbronchial Needle Aspiration in the Diagnostic Workup of Peripheral Lung Lesions. Lung. 2015;193;767-772.

2. Takai M, Izumo T, Chavez C, et al. Transbronchial needle aspiration through a guide sheath with endobronchial ultrasonography (GS-TBNA) for peripheral pulmonary lesions. Ann Thorac Cardiovasc Surg 2014;20:19-25.

3. Minezawa T, Okamura T, Yatsuya H, et al. Bronchus sign on thin-section computed tomography is a powerful predictive factor for successful transbronchial biopsy using endobronchial ultrasound with a guide sheath for small peripheral lung lesions: a retrospective observational study. BMC Med Imaging 2015;15:21.

Question I.28 Which of the following statements is TRUE?

A. cTBNA has a higher rate of bleeding or infectious complications than EBUS-TBNA.

B. cTBNA has a sensitivity that is equal to that of EBUS-TBNA for station 7 and 10 nodes.

C. EBUS-TBNA may cause metal particle contamination of sampled lymph nodes.

D. EBUS-TBNA has greater sensitivity than cTBNA for station 7 nodes larger than 2 cm.

Answer: C

Endobronchial ultrasound (EBUS) can be used to aspirate lymph nodes under real-time visual control with a very high sensitivity that exceeds 90%. Conventional transbronchial needle aspiration (cTBNA) has a diagnostic yield ranging from 36 to 84%, even with the use of rapid on-site evaluation (ROSE). Nevertheless, EBUS-TBNA provides little advantage over the cTBNA for lymph nodes that are more than 1.5 cm in size and are located in easy-to-access lymph node stations such as the subcarinal, paratracheal and hilar stations. EBUS-TBNA is safe and highly accurate for the diagnosis and staging of mediastinal and hilar lymph nodes in patients with known or suspected lung malignancy. Few complications of EBUS-TBNA are described in the medical literature. It has been reported that EBUS-TBNA needles may release metal particles, probably by friction between the stylet and the needle, with the potential risk of injecting metal particles into the nodes. The long-term consequences of this are unknown. As of this writing, there have been no studies of possible metal particle contamination after cTBNA.

References

1. Gounant V, Ninane V, Janson X, et al. Release of metal particles from needles used for transbronchial needle aspiration. Chest 2011;139:138-143.

2. Varela-Lema L, Fernández-Villar A, Ruano-Ravina A. Effectiveness and safety of endobronchial ultrasound-transbronchial needle aspiration: a systematic review. Eur Respir J 2009;33:1156-1164.

Question I.29 A 69 year old smoker female presented with cough, fever and weight loss. CT scan showed a left hilar mass with PET positive nodes at stations 10L and 4L. Flexible bronchoscopy is requested for diagnosis. You choose to:

A. Send the patient to another hospital because it is mandatory to sample multiple lymph nodes under EBUS guidance.

B. Initially perform cTBNA with ROSE on station 4R nodes because results will change the treatment approach.

C. Biopsy the tumor for diagnosis, then perform cTBNA of station 4L only because results will affect the treatment strategy.

D. Biopsy the central tumor using ROSE (rapid on site examination) because PET shows it to be unresectable. Lymph node sampling is not necessary.

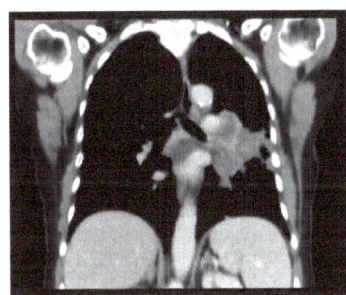 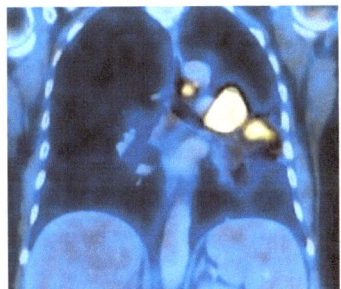 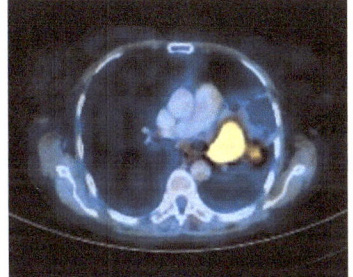

Answer: B

This patient likely has bronchogenic carcinoma. Although taking a direct biopsy of the left-sided tumor will make a diagnosis and likely assure adequate tissue for molecular testing, optimal patient management requires staging and thus a systematic lymph node sampling of possible N2 and N3 nodal stations is warranted. PET-CT suggests stage IIIA disease, but the presence of N1 nodes and of a central mass increases the likelihood of occult mediastinal involvement to as high as 20-25%. Furthermore, lung cancer patients with single N2 zone positivity have a significantly higher survival rate than patients with multiple N2 involvement and have a prognosis similar to patients with multiple positive N1 lymph nodes. If this patient has lung cancer, the extent of N2 disease or presence of N3 disease should be confirmed or ruled out before final therapeutic decisions are made. To address this query, EBUS-TBNA is likely warranted. as its yield for mediastinal staging is equivalent to mediastinoscopy when EBUS-TBNA is performed using a standardized approach (N3 nodes sampled first, then N2, then N1; sampling any lymph node greater than 5 mm in the short axis). In the absence of easy access to EBUS-TBNA, however, this patient can be managed using results from cTBNA and ROSE. We know the patient has a PET positive 4L lymph node. Overall, PET-CT positive predictive value is reportedly 63% and specificity is 88%. PET positive lymph nodes should be confirmed because PET positivity can be associated with postobstructive pneumonia, or be associated with infection, sarcoidosis, anthrocosis, or neoplasia. We also know that PET can be negative in involved nodes (the sensitivity of PET scanning for detecting mediastinal lymph node involvement is approximately 80%). Because the sensitivity of cTBNA is similar to that of EBUS-TBNA at station 4R, sampling this station by cTBNA and ROSE is a reasonable approach to diagnose N3 disease (if 4R nodes are positive the patient's tumor would be upstaged to stage IIIB, altering the treatment strategy.) If ROSE is used during cTBNA and station 4R is negative, then stations 7 and 4L (both N2 nodes) should be sampled next. The sensitivity of cTBNA is similar to that of EBUS-TBNA at station 7, though not quite as good as EBUS at station 4L. If samples from stations 4L (left lower paratracheal) or 7 (subcarinal) are positive, N2 disease would be confirmed, changing the surgical therapeutic approach to one of neoadjuvant therapy or definitive chemoradiation therapy. In addition to obtaining samples for diagnosis and optimizing diagnostic yield by using ROSE, sufficient tissue should be obtained for molecular analysis using proper aspiration and tissue processing techniques. This is increasingly relevant as targeted treatments continue to be developed and tissue requirements for comprehensive molecular testing (i.e. next generation sequencing) will likely continue to increase. High concordance in molecular tests between aspirates (e.g. cTBNA) and biopsies has been reported. Taking a direct biopsy of the left-sided tumor to make a diagnosis of cancer, without nodal sampling or sending specimens for molecular analysis would not be considered optimal patient management.

References

1. Herth F, Becker HD, Ernst A. Conventional vs endobronchial ultrasound-guided transbronchial needle aspiration: a randomized trial. Chest. 2004;125:322-325.

2. Diagnosis and management of Lung Cancer, 3º Ed: ACCP Guidelines. Chest 2013;143:e211S-50S.

3. Sun PL, Jin Y, Kim H, et al. High concordance of EGFR mutation status between histologic and corresponding cytologic specimens of lung adenocarcinomas. Cancer Cytopathol. 2013;121:311-319.

4. Munden RF, Swisher SS, Stevens CW et al. Imaging of the patient with non-small cell lung cancer. What the clinician wants to know. Radiology 2005;237:803-818.

5. Rami-Porta R, Crowley JJ, Goldstraw P. The revised TNM staging for lung cancer. Ann Thorac Cardiovasc Surg 2009;15:4-9.

Question I.30 Imagining the interior of the airway as a clock face and using the carina as the central reference point, transbronchial needle aspiration at approximately the 12 o'clock position along the anterior wall of the trachea at a level between the first and second intercartilaginous interspace from the lower trachea will sample:

A. The sub sub carina lymph node

B. The sub carina lymph node

C. The posterior carina lymph node

D. The anterior carina lymph node

Answer: D

If this seems confusing, do not be surprised. Until recently, lymph node mapping systems had different names, and sometimes, different descriptions. Nomenclatures included The Mountain system (named after famous MD Anderson thoracic surgeon Cliff Mountain), the Naruke system, the MD-ATS system, the WANG system, and the IASLC staging system. Today, for the most part, the world uses the IASLC lymph node map from the International Association for the Study of Lung Cancer. The descriptions provided in the above multiple choice selection are no longer used, and instead are referred to as simply level 7 lymph nodes. Follows, however, is an example of a detailed description: the anterior carina lymph node is in front and between the proximal portion of the right and left main bronchus on computed tomography scanning. It may be helpful to first lodge the needle tip into the mucosa, then to advance the needle catheter so that the entire length of the needle protrudes beyond the tip of the bronchoscope. One technique is for the bronchoscopist to anchor the proximal end of the catheter to the bronchoscope, preventing the needle from recoiling into the bronchoscope when resistance is encountered. The scope and the needle catheter can then be pushed simultaneously and as a single unit into the lesion. As the ensemble is advanced, the bronchoscope and catheter will curve slightly in a cephalad direction, moving the needle tip into a more perpendicular orientation at the puncture site. This helps avoid cartilaginous rings and also prompts a deeper insertion depth of the needle. By the way, in order to sample the posterior carina lymph node, the needle should be inserted at the posterior portion of the carina at about the 6 o'clock position.

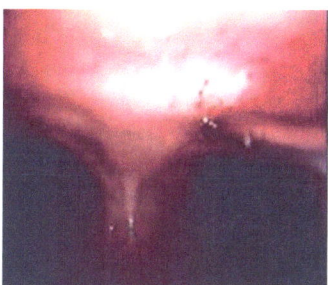

CONGRATULATIONS

You have now completed studying module I of The Essential cTBNA Bronchoscopist©.

You can now take the post-test for this module The following section contains a twelve question post-test and answers.

Post-tests are multiple-choice, single BEST answer. Please remember that while many programs consider 70% correct responses a passing grade, the student's "target" score should be 100%.

Please send us your opinion regarding Bronchoscopy Education Project materials by contacting your national bronchology association or emailing us at www.bronchoscopy.org.

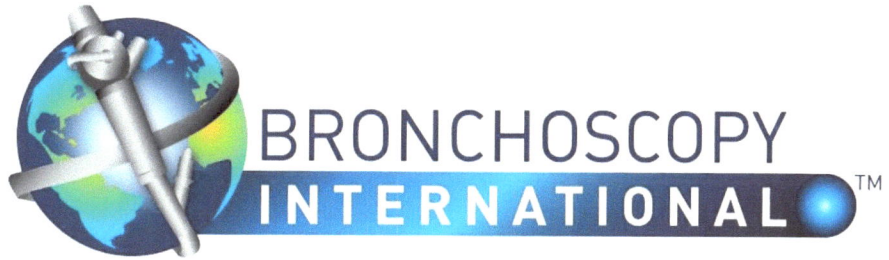

NOTES

The Essential cTBNA Bronchoscopist
Module I Post-test

Question 1. Which of the following statements about cTBNA sampling technique and smears is correct?

    A. Delayed sample processing may result in coagulation of material inside the needle.

    B. The quantity of sample fluid should be only a small drop.

    C. When excessive force is applied between slides, diagnostic material can be destroyed.

    D. Presence of bubbles on the slide can cause uneven distribution of sample material.

    E. All of the above.

Question 2. Which anatomic structure could be penetrated during conventional TBNA of a level 7 node?

    A. Azygos vein.

    B. Left brachiocephalic artery.

    C. Left atrium.

    D. Right atrium.

    E. Left ventricle.

Question 3. Which of the following statements is correct?

    A. Higher yields may be obtained by obtaining aspirates from the periphery of the node.

    B. Higher yields may be obtained by obtaining aspirates from the center of the node.

    C. Higher yields may be obtained by obtaining aspirates from the most heterogeneous part of the node.

    D. The yield is the same either by obtaining aspirates from the periphery, the center or the most heterogeneous part of the node.

Question 4. EBUS TBNA and conventional TBNA are of equal efficacy for sampling which of the following nodal stations?

    A. Station 10R

    B. Station 4L

    C. Station 7

    D. Station 5

Question 5. A small malignant endobronchial abnormality is noted in the bronchus intermedius 0.5 cm beyond the right upper lobe bronchial orifice. Transcarinal needle aspirations are positive. CT scans reveal no other organ involvement. Which of the following best describes this patient's clinical TNM stage?

    A. T3 N1 M0

    B. T3 N2 M0

    C. T2 N2 M0

    D. T1 N2 M0

    E. None of the above

Question 6. A transbronchial needle aspiration directed posteriorly and medially 1 cm beyond the origin of the right or left lower lobe bronchus risks entering which of the following?

    A. The pulmonary veins.

    B. The pulmonary arteries.

    C. The esophagus.

    D. The desccending aorta.

Question 7. Increased yield from transbronchial needle aspiration most likely results from:

    A. Multiple passes and on-site examination by an expert cytopathologist.

    B. Using the piggy-back nedle insertion technique.

    C. Applying suction while the needle is being removed from the lymph node.

    D. Using the jab or hub-against-the-wall insertion techniques.

Question 8. Each of the following is a well-described and acceptable name of a cTBNA technique EXCEPT:

A. Jabbing method.

B. Piggy-back method.

C. Cough method.

D. Hub-against-the-wall method.

E. Blind-insertion method.

Question 9. IASLC nodal station 4 R is accessed by:

A. Transbronchial needle aspiration 2-4 intercartilaginous spaces posterolateral to the trachea.

B. Transbronchial needle aspiration 2-4 intercartilaginous spaces anterolateral to the trachea.

C. Transbronchial needle aspiration 2-4 intercartilaginous spaces lateral to the trachea.

D. Transbronchial needle aspiration posterolateral to the trachea at the level of the carina.

Question 10. Which of the following anatomic structures lies immediately adjacent to the anterior wall of the left main bronchus and left upper lobe bronchus?

A. Left pulmonary artery.

B. Aorta.

C. Left pulmonary veins.

D. Esophagus.

Question 11. Transbronchial needle aspiration of IASLC station 7 is best performed by:

A. Inserting the needle in a relatively horizontal fashion against the medial wall of the right main bronchus across from and just proximal to the take off of the right upper lobe bronchus.

B. Inserting the needle in a relatively vertical fashion against the medial wall of the right main bronchus across from and just proximal to the take off of the right upper lobe bronchus.

C. Inserting the needle through the posterior wall of lower third of the trachea at the level of the carina.

Question 12. All of the following help prevent damage to the flexible bronchoscope during transbronchial needle aspiration EXCEPT:

A. Withdrawing the needle into its sheath before the sheath is withdrawn into the bronchoscope.

B. Straightening the bronchoscope before needle removal.

C. Good communiciation with your bronchoscopy assistants.

D. Avoiding excessive flexion or extension of the tip of the bronchoscope while the needle is passed through the working channel of the bronchoscope.

E. Avoiding use of the histology needle.

***

ANSWERS

TO MODULE 1, TWELVE QUESTION POST-TEST

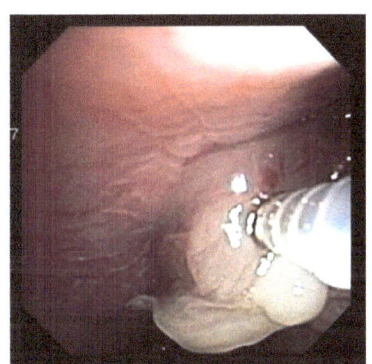 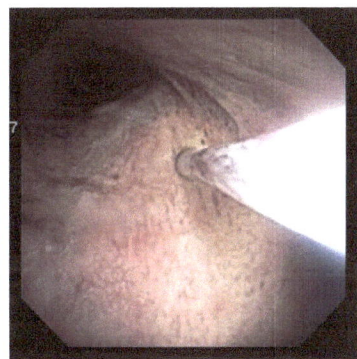

Answers to 12 question cTBNA Bronchoscopist post-test

ANSWERS

1. E
2. C
3. A
4. C
5. C
6. A
7. A
8. E
9. B
10. C
11. A
12. E

TOTAL SCORE _____/12

CONGRATULATIONS

You have now completed

The Essential Conventional TBNA Bronchoscopist

This is an important achievement on your journey to competency. We know that you will use what you have learned to enhance your bronchoscopy skills.

This reading assignment is complementary to other components of the Conventional TBNA curriculum, just one part in your quest to become a more competent and knowledgeable bronchoscopist.

We encourage you to attend national and international professional medical society meetings around the world so that you may share your experiences with your colleagues. We also urge you to explore the Bronchoscopy International website (www.bronchoscopy.org) for other learning materials, and to search instructional videos on the BronchOrg YouTube site. (See Video)

We look forward to receiving your comments regarding this and other components of The Bronchoscopy Education Project.

Please do not hesitate to contact your regional bronchology association, or email us at www.bronchoscopy.org

Thank you for participating in The Bronchoscopy Education Project!

§

CONTRIBUTORS

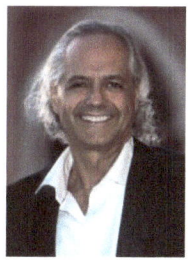 **Henri Colt M.D**. is Professor Emeritus with the University of California and an internationally recognized leadership coach and award winning medical educator. In addition to his lectures, academic achievements, leadership positions in professional medical societies, and travels to more than one hundred countries, he has published numerous articles and book chapters on all aspects of interventional pulmonology. As an expert in competency-oriented processes and procedures pertaining to bronchoscopy and other areas of pulmonary medicine, Colt has also served as a consultant to several large universities, governmental organizations, and national medical societies.

Dr. Septimiu Murgu is an Associate Professor of Pulmonary and Critical Care Medicine with the University of Chicago, and a certified Master Instructor with Bronchoscopy International. He has participated in Faculty Development programs in Singapore, Japan, India, Romania, and the United States. He is the coauthor of *The Essential EBUS Bronchoscopist* (Rake press), and of the popular textbook *Bronchoscopy and Central Airways Disorders: a patient-centered approach* (Elsevier press).

Dr. Nikos Koufos is a board certified Pulmonary and Critical Care physician in Athens, Greece with medical experiences in Romania, Spain, and the United States. He a certified Instructor with Bronchoscopy International and has participated in Faculty Development Programs in Greece, Romania, and Russia.

Dr. Grigoris Stratakos is an Associate Professor of Pulmonary Medicine and Head of the Interventional Pulmonology section (1st Respiratory Medicine Dept.) at Athens University Hospital in Greece. He is a certified Instructor with Bronchoscopy International and has participated in Faculty Development programs in Greece and Hungary.

Dr. Patricia Vujacich is Head of the Bronchoscopy Department at the Hopital de Clinicas in Buenos Aires, Argentina and a Master Instructor with Bronchoscopy International. She has spearheaded numerous training courses and other major bronchoscopy educational programs in South and Central America.

Dr. Hernan Iannella is a board certified Pulmonary physician and academic faculty at the Hopital de Clinicas in Buenos Aires, Argentina. He is also a certified Instructor with Bronchoscopy International.

§

The Essential Conventional TBNA Bronchoscopist© is the third of six volumes in The Essential Bronchoscopist™ Series. In addition to module-specific competency-oriented learning objectives and post-tests, it contains 30 multiple choice question/answer sets pertaining to conventional transbronchial needle aspiration (cTBNA). Topics include mediastinal anatomy, proper equipment handling, patient preparation, procedural indications contraindications and complications, bronchoscopic techniques, nodal sampling strategies, lung cancer staging and classification, specimen collection, processing, and expected results for diagnosing malignant and benign mediastinal disorders.

The aim of **The Essential Conventional TBNA Bronchoscopist**© is to prompt discussion among colleagues and to enrich the reader's experiential knowledge of this medical procedure*. Question/answer sets may be used in low-stakes continuing self-learning assessments, and to complement traditional apprenticeship style learning, thus contributing to the acquisition of cognitive and affective knowledge, as well as technical skill needed to become a competent Conventional TBNA bronchoscopist.

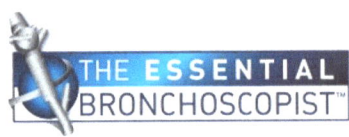

The Essential Bronchoscopist™ Series includes

- The Essential Flexible Bronchoscopist©
- The Essential EBUS Bronchoscopist©
- The Essential Conventional TBNA Bronchoscopist©
- The Essential Intensivist Bronchoscopist©
- The Essential Interventional Bronchoscopist©
- The Essentials of Bronchoscopy Education©

*The Essential Conventional TBNA Bronchoscopist is officially endorsed by numerous professional medical associations, and is a recommended reading assignment of the Bronchoscopy Education Project.

THE ESSENTIAL BRONCHOSCOPIST™ SERIES

Visit our website at
www.bronchoscopy.org

THE ESSENTIAL cTBNA BRONCHOSCOPIST©

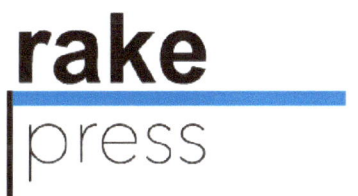

Laguna Beach, CA